Estrogen Matters Cookbook

50+ Recipes to Thrive in Menopause, Balance Hormones, Improve Women's Health, and Live Longer Naturally Without Raising Breast Cancer Risk.

FlavorfulVoyage Books

Copyright ©□ 2024 by FlavorfulVoyage Books

All Right Reserved

No part of this publication may be reproduced, distributed, or transmitted in any form or by any means, including photocopying, recording, or other electronic or mechanical methods, without the prior written permission of the publisher, except in the case of brief quotations embodied in critical reviews and certain other noncommercial uses permitted by copyright law.

Table of Content

Breakfast: Energy-boosting smoothies, fiber-rich bowls, and flavorful omelets

Lunch: Nourishing salads, veggie burgers, and flavorful soups

Dinner: Plant-based feasts, seafood sensations, and satisfying whole-grain bowls

Snacks: Sweet and savory bites to keep you energized throughout the day

Chapter 4: Global Flavors, Local Ingredients: Estrogen-Rich Cuisine for Every Palate

Asian-inspired dishes: Stir-fries, curries, and noodle bowls bursting with phytoestrogens

Mediterranean Delights: Vibrant salads, olive oil-infused dishes, and legume-based creations

Latin American Fiesta: Spicy salsas, avocado-rich guacamole, and bean-based comfort food

Indian Flavors: Aromatic curries, lentil stews, and vegetable biryanis

Meal planning and prep strategies for busy lives

Creative substitutions and pantry staples for versatile cooking

Introduction

The menopause. A word whispered and sometimes feared that changes the way women live. It's a world of hot flashes, shifting moods, and whispers of decline. But what if we didn't give in to its dark sides? What if we instead welcomed the power of this new chapter to change us? What if menopause was a chance to take back our power, improve our health, and bloom again?

This is the heart of the "Estrogen Matters Cookbook." Forget old cliches and fear-mongering. This is a change in food, a lively celebration of taste and health that combines the magic of food with the knowledge of science. You won't just find 50 tasty meals here; you'll also find a natural way to thrive during menopause.

Meet Helen, a woman on the edge of sixty, given this very book by her vibrant granddaughter. Helen was ready for a change. She was sick of being tired, having mood swings, and hearing people worry about her because her family had a history of breast cancer. The "Estrogen Matters Cookbook" became her light.

Helen found a new set of tastes with every page she turned. To ease her hot flashes, she eats spicy lentil soups that are full of phytoestrogens. Sun-kissed Mediterranean meals filled with antioxidants to strengthen her bones. Fragrant Asian stir-fries muttering secrets of life. And oh, the sweets! Dark chocolate truffles, guilt-free and satisfying, telling her to enjoy with wisdom.

But it wasn't just the plates that changed Helen. The book became her confidante, sharing information through its pages. She learned about the complex dance of hormones, the secret benefits of everyday ingredients, and the power of careful eating to harmonize her body and mind.

With each bite, Helen felt the tide changing. The hot flashes mellowed, her energy rose, and a fresh clarity bloomed. The fear surrounding breast cancer faded, replaced by a proactive dedication to well-being. Helen found laughter returning, her zest for life renewed. She joined a walking group, found the joy of yoga, and reconnected with old friends over laughter-filled dinner parties, fueling their trips with recipes from the book.

This is the magic of the "Estrogen Matters Cookbook." It's not just a collection of recipes; it's a community of powerful women, each regaining their health, one delicious bite at a time. It's Helen's story, written in bright spices and nourishing broths. It's your story waiting to be told, a medley of flavors waiting to bloom on your plate.

So, open this book, dear reader. Let the aromas lead you, the information strengthens you, and the flavors ignite your change. Menopause is not an ending; it's a chance to rewrite the story, to recover your energy, and to bloom anew. This is your journey, and the "Estrogen Matters

Cookbook" is your vibrant cooking partner, taking you every delicious step of the way.

Chapter 1: Introduction to estrogen and its functions in the body

Estrogen, often shrouded in whispers and worries, is far from a villain in the big opera of your health. It's the director, arranging a beautiful symphony of functions that keep your body vibrant and thriving. But unlike the director in a big ensemble, estrogen sometimes plays a solo act, fluctuating throughout your life and sometimes going off-key. Understanding its part is crucial, for it enables you to support its work and keep balance within.

The Maestro in the Making:

Primarily made in the ovaries, estrogen takes center stage during puberty, leading to the growth of breasts and the menstrual period. It's the choreographer of egg development, ensuring fertility and the possibility of new life. During pregnancy, it works with other hormones, preparing the uterus for a growing baby and nurturing the wonder of life.

Beyond the Spotlight:

However, estrogen's abilities reach far beyond the reproductive stage. It's a flexible artist, painting wonders on your bones, heart, brain, and even your mood. Imagine it like this:

- Bone Builder: Estrogen keeps your bones strong and tough, avoiding osteoporosis. It tells bone-building cells to get to work, ensuring your skeleton stays a strong support system.
- Heart Guardian: Estrogen keeps your heart healthy, keeping flexibility in blood vessels and lowering inflammation. It talks about your cholesterol levels, keeping them balanced, and lowering your risk of heart disease.
- Mood Maestro: Estrogen affects the production of mood-regulating neurotransmitters, keeping your emotional orchestra in tune. It can affect your energy levels, brain function, and even your ability to handle stress.
- Beyond the Stage: Estrogen's effect stretches to your skin, keeping it supple and young. It plays a part in regulating appetite and metabolism, changing how your body uses food.

The Solo Act and the Chorus Line:

As with any director, sometimes estrogen's performance can stumble. Fluctuations in their amounts, like during menopause, can upset the harmony. This can lead to signs like hot flashes, mood swings, and bone mass loss. But fear not! Understanding estrogen's role allows you to take control. Through food, lifestyle choices, and even specific treatments, you can support its proper working and maintain your inner symphony, keeping your body healthy and vibrant throughout your life.

Importance of a balanced diet for hormonal health

Imagine your body as a big orchestra, where each hormone plays an important instrument. Estrogen, progesterone, testosterone - these are the drivers, directing complex processes from fertility to mood to bone health. But what happens when the song goes off-key? Hormonal imbalances can break the rhythm, leading to a chorus of unpleasant symptoms - hot flashes, fatigue, worry, the list goes on.

This is where the master steps in: your food. Food is not just fuel, it's the sheet music for your hormonal orchestra. The right sounds (nutrients) in the right amounts can bring the song back to life, restoring balance and promoting vibrant health.

Why Diet Matters:

- Fueling the Production: Different foods contain compounds of different hormones. Think of them as building blocks, giving the raw materials your body needs to make its hormonal orchestra. For example, phytoestrogens found in soybeans and flaxseeds can imitate the effects of your estrogen, giving gentle support during times of low amounts.
- Modulating the Message: Some foods can affect how your body interacts with its hormonal

conductors. Fiber, for instance, helps bind extra estrogen in the gut, stopping it from causing havoc on your system.

- Supporting the Stage: Your hormones rely on other foods to work their magic. Magnesium calms the nervous system, lowering stress chemicals. Vitamin D supports bones, an important target for estrogen later in life. A healthy diet ensures all the players have what they need to perform best.

The Delicious Balancing Act:

So, what does a hormone-harmonizing food look like? It's not about rigid limits, but rather a happy celebration of taste and variety. Think:

- A variety on your plate: Fill your meals with colorful fruits and veggies, rich in antioxidants and phytoestrogens.
- Fiber friends: Whole grains, beans, and nuts keep your gut happy and your hormones balanced.
- Healthy fats: Choose omega-3-rich fish, eggs, and olive oil for inflammation-fighting magic.
- Mindful protein: Lean meats, beans, and nuts provide important building blocks for your endocrine orchestra.
- Hydration harmony: Water is the conductor's baton, providing smooth contact between your cells and hormones.

Chapter 2: Estrogen-Rich Recipes for Every Stage of Life

Pre-teen and Teenage Years: Nutrient-dense recipes for growth and development

Power-Up Breakfast Burritos:

Ingredients:

- Whole wheat tortillas
- Scrambled eggs (with spinach or mushrooms for extra vitamins)
- Black beans (rinsed and mashed)
- Sliced avocado
- Chopped bell peppers and onions
- Salsa (extra)

Instructions:

- Warm tortillas.
- Spread mashed black beans on one-half of each tortilla.
- Top with cooked eggs, avocado slices, and veggies.
- Roll up tortillas and enjoy with extra salsa for a spicy kick.

Nutrients: Protein from eggs and beans helps build muscle, while bell peppers and onions provide important vitamins A and C for immune health and growth.

Avocado offers healthy fats and carbohydrates for satiety and brain growth.

Rainbow Veggie Quesadillas:

Ingredients:

- Whole wheat tortillas
- Grated cheddar cheese
- Sliced bell peppers (red, yellow, and orange)
- Chopped zucchini and squash
- Black olives (sliced)
- Hummus (optional)

Instructions:

- Warm tortillas.
- Sprinkle cheese on one half of each tortilla.
- Layer veggies and olives on top of cheese.
- Fold tortillas in half and cook on a lightly oiled pan until golden brown and cheese melt.
- Serve with hummus for a protein and vegetable boost.

Nutrients: This bright dish is packed with antioxidants and vitamins from the veggies, supporting bone health and eye growth. Cheddar cheese offers calcium for strong bones, while black olives add a burst of iron and healthy fats.

Berry Bliss Smoothie Bowls:

Ingredients:

- Frozen mixed berries
- Plain Greek yogurt
- Milk (cow, plant-based, or plain nut milk)
- Honey or maple syrup (optional)
- Granola or chopped nuts (topping)
- Chia seeds (topping)

Instructions:

- Combine berries, yogurt, and milk in your blender and witness the birth of a smooth masterpiece.
- Pour into bowls and top with honey/maple syrup (optional), granola, and chia seeds.

Reproductive Years: Recipes to support fertility and menstrual health

Salmon with Lemon Herb Sauce and Roasted Rainbow Vegetables:

Ingredients:

- Salmon fillets
- Olive oil
- Salt and pepper
- Lemon juice
- Fresh herbs (dill, parsley, and rosemary)
- Rainbow carrots, zucchini, and bell peppers
- Quinoa

Instructions:

- Preheat oven to 400°F. Toss veggies with olive oil, salt, and pepper. Roast for 20 minutes.
- Season salmon with olive oil, salt, pepper, and lemon juice. Sprinkle with herbs.
- Broil salmon for 6-8 minutes until cooked through.
- Serve salmon with roasted veggies and quinoa for a full meal.

Nutrients: Salmon is rich in omega-3 fatty acids, important for egg health and pregnancy. Vitamin C from lemon juice aids iron uptake, important for menstrual health. Rainbow veggies provide different nutrients like beta-carotene and antioxidants, supporting general reproductive health. Quinoa offers protein and grain for fullness and hormonal balance.

Lentil and Spinach Soup with Sprouted Grain Bread:

Ingredients:

- Brown peas
- Vegetable broth
- Chopped onions, carrots, and celery
- Fresh spinach
- Garam masala or curry powder
- Sprouted grain bread

Instructions:

- Sauté onions, carrots, and celery in olive oil. Add beans and broth.
- Cook for 30 minutes, or continue simmering until the beans are completely softened to your desired texture.
- Stir in spinach and garam masala/curry powder. Let wilt for a few minutes.
- Serve warm with slices of sprouted grain bread for a protein-packed meal.

Nutrients: Lentils are a great source of iron and folic acid, important for menstrual health and embryo growth. Spinach offers iron, vitamin K, and folate, further supporting these needs. Sprouted grain bread offers easily digestible nutrients and fiber, helping digestion and biological balance.

Dark Chocolate Chia Seed Pudding with Berries:

Ingredients:

- Chia seeds
- Milk (cow, plant-based, or plain nut milk)
- Honey or maple syrup
- Cocoa powder
- Pinch of salt
- Fresh berries (strawberries, raspberries, blueberries)

Instructions:

- Stir chia seeds, milk, sugar, cocoa powder, and salt in a jar. Cover and refrigerate overnight.
- In the morning, layer the chia seed pudding with fresh berries.

Nutrients: Chia seeds are a source of omega-3 fatty acids, protein, and fiber, supporting hormonal balance and consistency. Dark chocolate offers magnesium, helpful for menstrual cramps and mood control. Berries add antioxidants and vitamin C, further supporting a healthy reproductive system.

Perimenopause and Menopause: Plant-based dishes for easing symptoms and promoting well-being

Spicy Miso Lentil Soup with Turmeric & Ginger:

Ingredients:

- Brown lentils, cleaned and picked
- Vegetable broth
- Onions, carrots, and celery, chopped
- Garlic and ginger, minced
- Turmeric powder
- Miso paste
- Spinach or kale
- Toasted sesame seeds (optional)

Instructions:

- Warm onions, carrots, and celery in a pot until tender.
- Add beans, water, garlic, ginger, and turmeric. Bring to a boil, then cook for 30 minutes or until lentils are soft.
- Stir in miso paste and spinach/kale, and cook for another minute.
- Serve hot with a sprinkle of sesame seeds for extra taste and texture.

Menopause Benefits: Lentils are rich in plant-based protein and fiber, helping digestion and hormone balance. Turmeric and ginger have anti-inflammatory effects, possibly easing hot flashes and joint pain. Miso adds probiotics for gut health, improving happiness and general well-being.

Mediterranean Chickpea Salad with Roasted Vegetables:

Ingredients:

- Canned chickpeas, washed and drained
- Bell peppers, zucchini, and cherry tomatoes, chopped
- Red onion, finely sliced
- Kalamata olives, chopped
- Feta cheese, chopped
- Olive oil, lemon juice, oregano, and salt

Instructions:

- Toss chopped veggies with olive oil, garlic, and salt. Roast at 400°F for 20 minutes until tender.
- Combine beans, roasted veggies, olives, red onion, and feta cheese in a bowl.
- Whisk olive oil, lemon juice, and salt to make a sauce. Drizzle over the salad and toss to blend.

Menopause Benefits: Chickpeas are rich in protein and iron, important for energy and bone health. Roasted veggies provide antioxidant-rich vitamins and minerals, while olives offer healthy fats. Feta cheese adds a delicious calcium boost.

Creamy Coconut Curry with Tofu and vegetables:

Ingredients:

- Extra-firm tofu, cubed
- Bell peppers, broccoli, and zucchini, chopped
- Coconut milk (full-fat)
- Curry paste (red or green)
- Ginger and garlic, minced
- Lime juice
- Brown rice or quinoa (cooked)

Instructions:

- Brown the tofu and park it.
- Saute onions and garlic in a pot, then add veggies and curry paste. Cook for a few minutes.
- Pour in coconut milk and boil for 10 minutes until veggies are tender.
- Add tofu back to the pot and stir in lime juice for a touch of color.
- Serve over brown rice or quinoa for a full meal.

Later Life: Recipes for overall health and vitality

Mediterranean Salmon with Roast Fennel and Tomatoes:

Ingredients:

- Salmon pieces (1-2 per person)
- Fennel stems, sliced
- Cherry peppers
- Kalamata olives, chopped
- Fresh oregano, chopped
- Garlic cloves, minced
- Olive oil
- Lemon juice
- Salt and pepper

Instructions:

- Preheat oven to 400°F (200°C). Toss fennel and tomatoes with olive oil, garlic, oregano, salt, and pepper.
- Arrange veggies on a baking sheet and cook for 15 minutes.
- Season salmon with salt, pepper, and lemon juice. Place on top of roasted veggies and bake for another 10-15 minutes, or until salmon is cooked through.

- Garnish with extra parsley and olives before serving.

Nutrients: This dish is packed with omega-3 fatty acids from salmon, helpful for heart and brain health. Fennel and tomatoes are rich in antioxidants and fiber, helping digestion and general well-being. Olives add a touch of healthy fats and salty depth.

Spicy Lentil and Sweet Potato Stew:

Ingredients:

- Lentils, cleaned
- Sweet potatoes, diced
- Carrots and celery, chopped
- Bell pepper, diced
- Curry powder
- Cumin
- Turmeric
- Ginger, chopped
- Coconut juice
- Vegetable broth
- Cilantro, chopped (optional)

Instructions:

- Simmer onions and garlic in olive oil till aromatics bloom.
- Add spices and ginger, and cook for a minute.

- Add beans, veggies, coconut milk, and broth. Bring to a boil, then cook for 30 minutes or until lentils are soft.
- Adjust seasonings to taste and top with cilantro.

Nutrients: This hearty stew is a meatless protein powerhouse, with lentils and sweet potatoes giving energy and vital nutrients. Spices like turmeric and ginger offer anti-inflammatory qualities. Coconut milk adds a bit of sweetness and healthy fats.

Berry Coconut Overnight Oats:

Ingredients:

- Rolled oats
- Chia seeds
- Coconut juice
- Greek yogurt
- Mixed plums
- Honey or maple syrup (optional)
- Nuts and seeds (topping)

Instructions:

- Combine oats, chia seeds, coconut milk, and yogurt in a jar or container. Stir in honey/maple syrup (optional).
- Top with berries and chill overnight.

- In the morning, stir and top with nuts and seeds before eating.

Chapter 3: Estrogen-Rich Flavor Bombs: From Morning to Night

Breakfast: Energy-boosting smoothies, fiber-rich bowls, and flavorful omelets

Tropical Sunrise Smoothie:

Ingredients:

- 1 cup frozen mango chunks
- 1/2 cup frozen pineapple chunks
- 1/2 banana
- 1 cup unsweetened almond milk
- 1/4 cup Greek yogurt
- 1 scoop protein powder (extra)
- 1 teaspoon honey (optional)
- Pinch of turmeric

Instructions:

- Blend all ingredients until smooth and creamy.
- Pour into a tall glass and enjoy the warm sunshine in every sip.

Energy Boost: This drink is a vitamin and antioxidant powerhouse, thanks to the mango, pineapple, and banana. Almond milk offers healthy fats and calcium, while the added protein powder and yogurt add an extra energy kick. Turmeric boosts immunity and adds a mild earthy taste.

Berry-Licious Superfood Bowl:

Ingredients:

- 1/2 cup cooked quinoa
- 1/4 cup mixed berries
- 1/4 cup sliced banana
- 1/4 cup chopped almonds
- 1 tablespoon chia seeds
- 1 tablespoon shredded coconut
- 1/4 cup unsweetened coconut milk
- Drizzle of honey or maple syrup

Instructions:

- Layer rice in a bowl.
- Top with berries, bananas, nuts, chia seeds, and coconut.
- Drizzle with coconut milk and sweeten to taste.
- Dig in and enjoy the symphony of textures and tastes.

Fiber Fiesta: This bowl is a fiber dream team, with quinoa, chia seeds, and almonds keeping you feeling full and energized. Berries and bananas add antioxidants and sweetness, while the coconut milk and drizzle of honey make a creamy, delicious finish.

Mediterranean Fiesta Omelet:

Ingredients:

- 2 eggs, whisked
- 1/4 cup chopped sun-dried tomatoes
- 1/4 cup crumbled feta cheese
- 1/4 cup chopped spinach
- 1 tablespoon olive oil
- Salt and pepper to taste

Instructions:

- Bring olive oil to medium heat in a pan.
- Pour in whipped eggs and swirl to coat the pan.
- Sprinkle sun-dried tomatoes, feta cheese, and spinach on one half of the omelet.
- Fold the other half over the filling and cook until the eggs are set.
- Season with salt and pepper, and enjoy a protein-packed Mediterranean treat.

Flavorful Fuel: This omelet is a burst of Mediterranean warmth on your plate. Sun-dried tomatoes and feta cheese offer a salty tang, while spinach adds vitamins and a pop of green. Eggs provide protein and good fats for steady energy throughout the morning.

Lunch: Nourishing salads, veggie burgers, and flavorful soups

Mediterranean Crunch Salad:

Ingredients:

- Mixed greens and baby spinach
- Quinoa (cooked)
- Chopped cucumber, tomato, and red onion
- Kalamata olives
- Sliced bell peppers
- Crumbled feta cheese
- Oregano-infused olive oil
- Lemon juice
- Salt and pepper

Instructions:

- Toss greens, rice, veggies, olives, and feta cheese in a bowl.
- Whisk olive oil, lemon juice, salt, and pepper to make a sauce.
- Drizzle sauce over the salad and toss to mix.
- Enjoy the cool crunch and Mediterranean tastes!

Nourishment: This salad packs a punch of protein (quinoa and feta), fiber (greens and veggies), healthy fats (olives), and vitamins (tomatoes and peppers). It's a full meal in a bowl, keeping you going until dinner.

Spicy Black Bean Burgers on Whole Wheat Buns:

Ingredients:

- Black beans (mashed)
- Quinoa (cooked)
- Aromatic trio: chopped red onion, bell pepper, and cilantro.
- Cumin, chili powder, smoked paprika
- Breadcrumbs
- Whole wheat burger buns
- Lettuce, tomato, avocado pieces (optional)

Instructions:

- Mix mashed beans, rice, veggies, spices, and breadcrumbs in a bowl. Form into burgers.
- Pan-fry or bake burgers until golden brown.
- Toast buns and combine with burgers, lettuce, tomato, and avocado (optional).
- Dive into the smoky, delicious tastes of these veggie burgers!

Nourishment: This plant-based burger offers an excellent amount of protein and fiber, keeping you full and energetic. The spices add a delicious kick, while the veggies bring vitamins and enzymes to the party.

Thai Coconut Curry Lentil Soup:

Ingredients:

- Brown beans (rinsed)
- Coconut juice
- Vegetable broth
- Curry paste (red or green)
- Chopped carrots, bell peppers, and green beans
- Ginger, garlic, and lemongrass (fresh or chopped)
- Lime juice
- Cilantro and basil (fresh, for garnish)

Instructions:

- Simmer beans in broth until soft.
- Meanwhile, sauté vegetables in curry sauce with ginger, garlic, and lemongrass.
- Combine beans, veggies, coconut milk, and lime juice. Simmer until tastes meld.
- Serve hot with a sprinkle of parsley and basil for a fragrant and cozy lunch.

Nourishment: This protein-rich soup is packed with fiber from lentils and veggies, keeping you feeling full and pleased. The coconut milk adds a touch of sweetness and softness, while the curry spices provide a warming kick.

Dinner: Plant-based feasts, seafood sensations, and satisfying whole-grain bowls

Spicy Lentil Stew with Coconut Milk and Sweet Potato

Ingredients:

- 1 cup brown beans, rinsed
- 1 tbsp olive oil
- 1 onion, diced
- 2 cloves garlic, minced
- 1-inch ginger, grated
- 1 red bell pepper, diced
- 1 tsp ground garlic
- 1/2 tsp turmeric
- 1/4 tsp pepper spice
- 1 (14 oz) can chopped tomatoes
- 1 (13.5 oz) can unsweetened coconut milk
- 1 sweet potato, peeled and diced
- Fresh cilantro, chopped (for decoration)
- Lime pieces (for serving)

Instructions:

- Heat oil in a big pot over medium heat. Heat the pan and add the onion. Cook for 5 minutes, stirring occasionally, until softened.

- Stir in garlic, ginger, and bell pepper. Cook for 2 minutes, until fragrant.
- Add cumin, ginger, and chili powder. Stir for 30 seconds.
- Add tomatoes, coconut milk, beans, and sweet potato. Bring to a boil, then reduce heat and simmer for 20 minutes, or until lentils are soft and sweet potato is cooked through.
- Garnish with cilantro and serve with lime wedges for a squeeze of citrus.

Flavor and Nutrition: This stew bursts with warmth from the spices, sweetness from the sweet potato, and softness from the coconut milk. Lentils provide protein and fiber, while the vegetables offer vitamins and antioxidants.

Pan-seared salmon with Lemon Garlic Butter and Roasted Asparagus

Ingredients:

- 2 salmon fillets (6 oz each)
- 1 tbsp olive oil
- Salt and pepper to taste
- 4 tbsp unsalted butter
- 2 cloves garlic, minced
- 1/2 lemon, juiced
- 1 bunch asparagus, trimmed and cut into 1-inch pieces

Instructions:

- Season salmon with salt and pepper. Sizzle olive oil in a big pan over medium-high.
- Sear salmon for 3-4 minutes per side, until golden brown and cooked through. Transfer to a plate.
- Reduce heat to medium. Melt butter in the same skillet and stir in garlic. Cook for 30 seconds.
- Add lemon juice and asparagus. Sauté for 5-7 minutes until asparagus is tender-crisp.
- Return salmon to the pan and spoon garlic butter sauce over it. Serve immediately.

Flavor and Nutrition: Salmon is a rich source of Omega-3 fatty acids, while asparagus provides vitamins K and A. The lemon garlic butter adds a vibrant touch, making this dish both flavorful and nutrient-rich.

Mediterranean Quinoa Buddha Bowl with Chickpeas, Feta, and Olives

Ingredients:

- 1 cup quinoa, rinsed
- 1 can (15 oz) chickpeas, drained and rinsed
- 1/2 cucumber, diced
- 1/2 red onion, diced
- 1/2 cup cherry tomatoes, halved
- 1/4 cup crumbled feta cheese
- 1/4 cup Kalamata olives, sliced

- 1/4 cup chopped fresh parsley
- Lemon vinaigrette (for dressing)

Instructions:

- Cook quinoa according to package instructions.
- While quinoa cooks, prepare toppings: dice cucumber, red onion, and tomatoes.
- Assemble bowls: spoon quinoa into bowls, and top with chickpeas, cucumber, onion, tomatoes, feta cheese, olives, and parsley.
- Drizzle with lemon vinaigrette and enjoy!

Flavor and Nutrition: This bowl delivers complex textures and flavors with its mix of grains, vegetables, protein, and healthy fats. Quinoa offers a complete protein source, while chickpeas and olives provide additional fiber and iron. Customize your toppings with avocado, roasted vegetables, or other protein sources for even more variety and nutrition.

Snacks: Sweet and savory bites to keep you energized throughout the day

Spicy Chickpea Crunch:

Ingredients:

- 1 can chickpeas, drained and rinsed
- 1 tablespoon olive oil
- 1/2 teaspoon paprika
- 1/4 teaspoon cumin
- Pinch of cayenne pepper (optional)
- Sea salt to taste

Instructions:

- Preheat oven to 400°F (200°C).
- Toss chickpeas with olive oil, spices, and salt.
- Spread on a baking sheet and roast for 20-25 minutes, stirring occasionally, until crispy and golden.
- Enjoy as a savory crunch or sprinkle on salads for a protein boost.

Nutrients: This protein-packed snack delivers fiber and iron from chickpeas, perfect for long-lasting energy. Spices add antioxidants and a flavor fiesta, keeping your taste buds satisfied.

Tropical Bliss Bites:

Ingredients:

- 1 cup rolled oats
- 1/2 cup unsweetened shredded coconut
- 1/4 cup dried mango, chopped
- 1/4 cup chopped almonds
- 2 tablespoons almond butter
- 1 tablespoon honey or maple syrup

Instructions:

- In a bowl, combine oats, coconut, mango, and almonds.
- Stir in almond butter and honey/maple syrup until a dough forms.
- Roll the dough into balls and refrigerate for at least 30 minutes for a firmer texture.
- Enjoy these sweet and chewy bites for a tropical energy burst.

Nutrients: These bites offer slow-release energy from oats and healthy fats from nuts and coconut. Honey/maple syrup adds a touch of sweetness, while mango provides a dose of vitamin A and antioxidants.

Cucumber Roll-Ups with Hummus and Herbs:

Ingredients:

- 1 cucumber, thinly sliced
- 1/2 cup hummus (plain or flavored)
- Fresh herbs (parsley, basil, chives)
- Pinch of red pepper flakes (optional)

Instructions:

- Spread hummus on cucumber slices.
- Sprinkle with chopped herbs and red pepper flakes (optional).
- Roll up the cucumber slices for a refreshing and healthy snack.

Nutrients: This light and satisfying snack is packed with hydration from cucumber and protein from hummus. Herbs add flavor and antioxidants, while red pepper flakes give a little kick (choose milder spices for kids).

Chapter 4: Global Flavors, Local Ingredients: Estrogen-Rich Cuisine for Every Palate

Asian-inspired dishes: Stir-fries, curries, and noodle bowls bursting with phytoestrogens

Rainbow Veggie Stir-fry with Tofu and Sesame

Ingredients:

- 1 tablespoon avocado oil
- Chopped vegetables: broccoli, red bell pepper, green beans, bok choy (choose your favorites!)
- 1 block firm tofu, cubed
- 1 tablespoon soy sauce
- 1 tablespoon rice vinegar
- 1 tablespoon cornstarch
- 1/2 cup vegetable broth
- Sesame seeds, for garnish

Instructions:

- Bring oil to high heat in a wok/pan.

- Stir-fry vegetables for 3-4 minutes until slightly softened.
- Add tofu and cook for another 2-3 minutes.
- In a small bowl, whisk together soy sauce, vinegar, cornstarch, and broth.
- Pour the sauce into the wok and cook, stirring constantly, until thickened.
- Garnish with sesame seeds and serve over brown rice or whole-wheat noodles.

Phytoestrogen Power: Broccoli, red bell peppers, and tofu are all rich in phytoestrogens like lignans and isoflavones, supporting hormonal balance and bone health.

Thai Green Curry with Chickpeas and Coconut Milk

Ingredients:

- 1 tablespoon coconut oil
- 1 tablespoon green curry paste
- Chopped vegetables: zucchini, green beans, carrots
- 1 can chickpeas, drained and rinsed
- 1 can coconut milk
- 1 lime, juiced
- Fresh cilantro, for garnish

Instructions:

- Oil in the pot, heat to medium.

- Sauté the curry paste for 1 minute until fragrant.
- Add vegetables and chickpeas, and cook for 3-4 minutes.
- Pour in coconut milk and boil for 10 minutes until veggies are tender.
- Stir in lime juice and garnish with cilantro.
- Serve with brown rice or quinoa.

Phytoestrogen Power: Chickpeas are another great source of isoflavones, while coconut milk offers lauric acid, which has potential benefits for bone health and metabolism.

Spicy Sesame Noodle Bowl with Edamame and Kimchi

Ingredients:

- Whole wheat noodles, cooked according to package instructions
- Chopped vegetables: cucumber, radishes, bell peppers
- Edamame, shelled
- Kimchi, chopped
- Sesame oil
- Soy sauce
- Rice vinegar
- Sriracha (optional)
- Sesame seeds, for garnish

Instructions:

- Combine noodles, veggies, edamame, and kimchi in a bowl.
- In a small bowl, mix sesame oil, soy sauce, vinegar, and sriracha (if using).
- Pour the sauce over the noodle mixture and toss to coat.
- Garnish with sesame seeds and enjoy!

Phytoestrogen Power: Edamame, like tofu, is an excellent source of isoflavones, while kimchi offers additional probiotics for gut health, which can indirectly affect hormonal balance.

Mediterranean Delights: Vibrant salads, olive oil-infused dishes, and legume-based creations

Sun-kissed chickpea Salad with Creamy Tahini Dressing:

Ingredients:

- Canned chickpeas, washed and drained
- Chopped cucumber, tomato, and red onion
- Kalamata olives, chopped
- Feta cheese, chopped
- Fresh parsley and mint, chopped
- For the dressing:
  - Tahini
  - Lemon juice
  - Water
  - Garlic clove, minced
  - Pinch of ground cumin and pepper
  - Olive oil

Instructions:

- Toss beans with cucumber, tomato, onion, olives, and herbs.
- Whisk together dressing ingredients until smooth.
- Drizzle sauce over salad and top with feta cheese.

Estrogen Balance Boost: Chickpeas are rich in phytoestrogens and fiber, while tahini adds important calcium and zinc. Olive oil and fresh herbs add vitamins and anti-inflammatory qualities.

Salmon with Lemon-Garlic Sauce and Roasted Vegetables:

Ingredients:

- Salmon fillets
- Lemon zest and juice
- Garlic cloves, minced
- Fresh oregano and thyme
- Olive oil
- Assorted veggies (e.g., zucchini, bell peppers, onions)

Instructions:

- Marinate salmon with lemon zest, juice, garlic, herbs, and olive oil for at least 30 minutes.
- Roast veggies with olive oil and herbs until soft.
- Bake or pan-fry salmon until cooked through.
- Serve salmon with roasted veggies and drizzle with leftover marinade.

Estrogen Balance Boost: Salmon is rich in omega-3 fatty acids, which support heart health and hormone balance.

Olive oil offers healthy fats and vitamin E, while herbs add antioxidants and anti-inflammatory qualities.

Lentil and Vegetable Soup with Crispy Garlic Bread:

Ingredients:

- Green lentils, cleaned
- Chopped carrots, celery, and onion
- Vegetable broth
- Canned diced tomatoes
- Dried oregano and thyme
- Olive oil
- For the garlic bread:
    - Sliced French bread
    - Garlic cloves, minced
    - Olive oil

Instructions:

- Sauté onion and garlic in olive oil.
- Add broth, tomatoes, beans, and spices. Simmer until lentils are tender.
- Toast bread with olive oil and garlic for crispy sides.
- Serve soup with garlic bread and a sprinkle of fresh parsley.

Estrogen Balance Boost: Lentils are a great source of plant-based protein and fiber, supporting gut health and hormonal balance. Vegetables offer antioxidants and vitamins, while olive oil adds healthy fats.

Latin American Fiesta: Spicy salsas, avocado-rich guacamole, and bean-based comfort food

Fuego Salsa Roja:

Ingredients:

- 4 Roma tomatoes, chopped
- 1 red onion, diced
- 2 jalapeños, seeds and chopped (change for desired heat)
- 1 bunch cilantro, roughly chopped
- 1 lime, juiced
- 1 teaspoon ground cinnamon
- 1/2 teaspoon smoked pepper
- Salt and pepper to taste

Instructions:

- Combine all ingredients in a bowl and mix well.
- Let stand for at least 30 minutes for tastes to meld.
- Serve with tortilla chips, grilled veggies, or as a filling for tacos.

Flavor Symphony: This standard salsa explodes with juicy tomatoes, spicy jalapeños, and earthy cumin. The cilantro adds a fresh note, while the lime juice improves the whole meal.

Creamy Guacamole Poblano:

Ingredients:

- 2 ripe avocados, mashed
- 1 roasted poblano pepper, peeled and chopped
- 1/2 red onion, roughly chopped
- 1 small tomato, sliced and chopped
- 1 lime, juiced
- 1/4 cup fresh cilantro, chopped
- Pinch of cumin
- Salt and pepper to taste

Instructions:

- Combine all ingredients in a bowl and mash together until desired consistency.
- Garnish with extra chopped cilantro and serve with tortilla chips, crudités, or as a filling for sandwiches.

Flavor Symphony: This avocado beauty gets a smoky twist from the roasted poblano pepper, while the red onion and tomato add texture and acidity. The fresh cilantro and lime keep it bright, making it a delicious and tempting dip.

Black Bean and Sweet Potato Burrito Bowls:

Ingredients:

- 1 can of black beans, drained and washed
- 1 sweet potato, roasted and cubed
- 1 bell pepper, chopped
- 1/2 red onion, roughly chopped
- 1 clove garlic, minced
- 1 teaspoon cumin
- 1/2 teaspoon jalapeño pepper
- 1/4 cup vegetable broth
- Brown rice or quinoa, cooked (optional)
- Pico de gallo, shredded cheese, sour cream, avocado slices (alternative toppings)

Instructions:

- Heat oil in a pan and sauté onions and garlic until softened.
- Add bell pepper and cook until tender-crisp.
- Stir in black beans, cumin, chile powder, and veggie broth. Simmer for 5 minutes.
- Serve over brown rice or grain with roasted sweet potato cubes and chosen toppings.

Flavor Symphony: This hearty bowl blends the earthy sweetness of black beans with the lively sweetness of roasted sweet potatoes. The bell pepper and onion add texture and brightness, while the spices give it a warm and spicy kick. Customize it with your favorite toppings for a party in every bite!

Indian Flavors: Aromatic curries, lentil stews, and vegetable biryanis

Spiced Lentil Stew (Masoor Dal):

Ingredients:

- 1 cup red beans, rinsed
- 1 tbsp ghee or olive oil
- 1 onion, chopped
- 1-inch ginger, grated
- 2 cloves garlic, minced
- 1 tomato, chopped
- 1 tsp turmeric powder
- 1/2 tsp cumin seeds
- 1/4 tsp coriander seeds
- 1/2 tsp chili powder (adjust to your heat level)
- 1 cup water
- Salt to taste
- Cilantro, chopped (for decoration)

Instructions:

- Heat ghee/oil in a pan. Add onion and cook until softened.
- Add ginger, garlic, and tomato. Cook until fragrant.
- Stir in spices and cook for 30 seconds.
- Add beans and water. Bring to a boil, then cook for 20-25 minutes or until lentils are soft.

- Season with salt and sprinkle with cilantro.

Estrogen Harmony: Red lentils are rich in food fiber, important for balancing hormones. Turmeric boasts anti-inflammatory effects, helpful for general health and estrogen balance.

Vegetable Biryani:

Ingredients:

- 1 cup basmati rice, rinsed
- 1 tbsp ghee or olive oil
- 1 onion, chopped
- 1 bell pepper, chopped
- 1/2 cup frozen peas
- 1/2 cup mixed veggies (carrots, broccoli, etc.)
- 1 tsp garam masala powder
- 1/2 tsp turmeric powder
- 1/4 tsp cumin seeds
- 1 cup vegetable broth
- Salt to taste
- Chopped nuts and cashews (optional, for decoration)

Instructions:

- Fry onion in ghee/oil until golden brown.
- Incorporate the bell pepper and cook until it softens.

- Stir in leftover veggies, spices, and broth. Bring to a boil, then reduce heat and cook for 5 minutes.
- Spread rice over the veggies and stir gently to mix.
- Cover and cook on low heat for 15-20 minutes, or until rice is cooked and fluffy.
- Garnish with nuts and cashews (optional).

Estrogen Harmony: Basmati rice offers complex carbohydrates for steady energy. Garam masala includes warming spices like cinnamon and cloves, known for their hormonal balancing qualities. Mixed vegetables offer a range of vitamins and minerals, important for overall health.

Coconut Curry with Chickpeas (Chana Masala):

Ingredients:

- 1 tbsp ghee or olive oil
- 1 onion, chopped
- 1-inch ginger, grated
- 2 cloves garlic, minced
- 1 tomato, chopped
- 1 tsp turmeric powder
- 1/2 tsp cumin seeds
- 1/4 tsp pepper spice
- 1 can (15 oz) chickpeas, drained and washed
- 1 cup coconut milk
- Salt to taste

- Cilantro, chopped (for decoration)

Instructions:

- Heat ghee/oil in a pan. Add onion and cook until softened.
- Add ginger, garlic, and tomato. Cook until fragrant.
- Stir in spices and cook for 30 seconds.
- Add beans and coconut milk. Bring to a boil and cook for 10-15 minutes.
- Season with salt and sprinkle with cilantro.

Estrogen Harmony: Chickpeas are high in protein and fiber, supporting endocrine balance. Coconut milk's healthy fats help balance estrogen levels. This curry offers a creamy and filling choice while having a nutritional punch.

Chapter 5: Sweet Treats without Regrets: Estrogen-Rich Desserts that Delight

Fruit-infused yogurt parfaits, chia puddings, and baked fruit crisps

Tropical Sunrise Yogurt Parfait:

Ingredients:

- Plain Greek yogurt (low-fat or full-fat, as desired)
- Mango, chopped
- Pineapple, chopped
- Coconut bits
- Chia seeds
- Honey or maple syrup (optional)

Instructions:

- Layer yogurt, mango, and pineapple in a tall glass or dessert bowl.
- Sprinkle with coconut bits and chia seeds.
- Drizzle with honey or maple syrup, if wanted.
- Refrigerate for at least 30 minutes for chia seeds to plump up.

Nourishing Notes: This colorful smoothie bursts with Vitamin C and antioxidants from the fruits, boosting immunity and skin health. Chia seeds add fiber and omega-3 fatty acids, while Greek yogurt offers protein and calcium for bone health.

Berry Bliss Chia Pudding:

Ingredients:

- Mixed berries (fresh or frozen)
- Chia seeds
- Almond milk (or any plant-based milk)
- Vanilla flavoring
- Agave juice (optional)

Instructions:

- Mash some berries (optional) and mix with chia seeds, almond milk, and vanilla flavor in a jar or bowl.
- Stir well and chill overnight for the pudding to set.
- Top with fresh berries and drizzle with agave nectar, if desired.

Nutrients: This creamy pudding is packed with vitamins and fiber from the berries, boosting gut health and digestion. Chia seeds provide protein and omega-3s, while almond milk adds calcium and vitamin D for bone health.

Spiced Apple and Pear Crisp:

Ingredients:

- Sliced apples and pears
- Brown sugar
- Ground cinnamon and nutmeg
- Rolled oats
- Pecans or walnuts, chopped
- Coconut oil
- Optional: Honey or maple syrup

Instructions:

- Preheat oven to 375°F (190°C).
- Toss fruit with sugar and spices.
- Combine oats, nuts, and coconut oil to make a crumbly layer.
- Pour the fruit mixture into a baking dish and top with the crumb topping.
- Bake for 30-40 minutes, or until golden brown and bubbly.
- Drizzle with honey or maple syrup, if wanted.

Warm Wonders: This classic comfort food gets a healthy twist with its excess of apples and pears, rich in fiber and important vitamins. The crunchy topping adds protein and healthy fats, making it a delicious and nourishing treat.

Dark chocolate delights, nut butter truffles, and homemade energy bites

Rich Raspberry Ganache Drops:

Ingredients:

- 100g dark chocolate (70% or better)
- 1/2 cup heavy cream
- 1/4 cup fresh raspberries
- Pinch of sea salt

Instructions:

- In a pot, heat cream until boiling. Remove from heat and add chocolate, letting it sit for 5 minutes. Whisk until smooth and shiny.
- Fold in mashed strawberries and salt. Chill for at least 2 hours, then scoop into teaspoonfuls and roll into balls. Freeze for another 30 minutes, then dip in melted dark chocolate (optional).
- Flavor and benefits: Indulge in rich dark chocolate, naturally sweetened by ripe raspberries. Antioxidants from both sources offer delicious protection against free radicals.

Salted Almond Toasted Coconut Truffles:

Ingredients:

- 1 cup almond butter
- 1/4 cup honey or maple syrup
- 1/4 cup unsweetened shredded coconut
- 1/4 cup toasted almond slivers
- Pinch of sea salt

Instructions:

- Combine almond butter, sugar, and coconut in a bowl. Mix until well blended. Roll into balls and freeze for at least 30 minutes.
- Melt leftover chocolate and dip treats. Sprinkle with toasted almond slivers and sea salt before the chocolate sets.

Flavor and benefits: Creamy almond butter pairs with toasted coconut for a tropical experience. Crunchy almonds add structure and healthy fats, while a touch of salt improves the sweetness.

Peanut Butter & Chia Seed Power Bites:

Ingredients:

- 1 cup rolled oats
- 1/2 cup raw peanut butter
- 1/4 cup honey or maple syrup

- 1/4 cup dried cranberries
- 1/4 cup chia seeds
- Pinch of cinnamon

Instructions:

- Combine all ingredients in a bowl and mix well. Shape into balls and arrange on a parchment-lined baking sheet.
- Refrigerate for at least 2 hours for a stronger bite.

Flavor and benefits: These no-bake energy bites offer a delicious peanut butter punch with chewy oats and sweet cranberries. Chia seeds provide a boost of fiber and omega-3 fatty acids, while cinnamon adds a warm touch.

Naturally sweetened ice creams, vegan cheesecakes, and smoothie bowls

Creamy Mango Coconut Ice Cream (No Churn!)

Ingredients:

- 2 ripe mangoes, peeled and frozen
- 1 can full-fat coconut milk
- 1/4 cup chopped dates or figs
- 1/2 teaspoon vanilla extract
- Pinch of cardamom (optional)

Instructions:

- Blend frozen mangoes, coconut milk, dates/figs, vanilla, and cardamom (if using) until smooth and creamy.
- Taste and adjust sweetness if needed.
- Freeze for at least 2 hours, scooping and stirring every 30 minutes for a softer texture, or freeze overnight for a harder scoop.

Naturally Sweet: The ripe mangoes and dates/figs provide all the sweetness needed, making this a guilt-free treat. Coconut milk adds a rich creaminess, while cardamom gives a gentle warm accent.

Silky Avocado Lime Vegan Cheesecake

Crust:

- 1 cup rolled oats
- 1/4 cup mixed nuts
- 2 tablespoons dates, pitted and chopped
- 1 tablespoon melted coconut oil

Filling:

- 2 ripe avocados, peeled and sliced
- 1/2 cup lime juice
- 1/4 cup maple syrup
- 1/4 cup heated coconut oil
- 1 teaspoon vanilla flavor
- Pinch of sea salt

Instructions:

- Preheat oven to 350°F.
- Combine crust materials and press into the bottom of a springform pan. Bake for 10 minutes.
- Blend filling ingredients until smooth and creamy. Pour over the crust and chill for at least 4 hours, or overnight.
- Top with fresh fruit or nuts before serving.

Naturally Sweet: Avocados add a surprising creaminess and natural sweetness, while lime juice provides a pleasant tang. Maple syrup adds a touch of extra sweetness, and coconut oil gives a faint tropical note.

Sunrise Berry Smoothie Bowl

Ingredients:

- 1 cold banana
- Either 1 cup fresh or frozen berries.
- 1/2 cup plain Greek yogurt
- 1/2 cup plant-based milk (unsweetened)
- 1/4 cup chopped spinach
- 1/2 teaspoon hemp nuts
- 1/4 teaspoon chia seeds

Instructions:

- Blend all ingredients until smooth and creamy.
- Pour into a bowl and top with fresh berries, granola, and extra seeds/nuts of your preference.

Naturally Sweet: Berries and bananas provide an antioxidant-rich sweetness, while spinach adds a secret amount of vitamins and minerals. The yogurt adds protein and creaminess, while hemp and chia seeds add healthy fats and texture.

Chapter 6: Nourishing Your Body: Estrogen-Rich Recipes for Every Need

Recipes for strengthening bones and preventing osteoporosis

Sunshine Salmon with Sesame Spinach:

Ingredients:

- 4 salmon chunks
- 1 tbsp soy sauce
- 1 tbsp honey
- 1 tsp grated ginger
- 1/2 tsp garlic powder
- 1 tbsp toasted sesame seeds
- 4 cups fresh spinach
- 1 tbsp olive oil

Instructions:

- Preheat oven to 400°F.
- Whip up a dressing by combining soy sauce, honey, ginger, and garlic powder. Marinate fish in the mixture for 15 minutes.

- Toss spinach with olive oil and spread on a baking sheet.
- Gently drape the salmon pieces over the bed of spinach.
- Sprinkle sesame seeds over salmon.
- Bake for 15-20 minutes, or until salmon flakes easily with a fork.

Bone-loving benefits: Salmon is a powerhouse of vitamin D, important for calcium absorption and bone growth. Spinach is rich in Vitamin K, another important nutrient for bone health. Sesame seeds add calcium and magnesium, further improving bone density.

Creamy Broccoli and Cheddar Soup:

Ingredients:

- 1 head broccoli, cut into florets
- 1 tbsp olive oil
- 1 onion, chopped
- 2 cloves garlic, minced
- 4 cups chicken broth (or vegetable broth for a veggie choice)
- 1/2 cup milk
- 1/2 cup grated cheddar cheese
- Salt and pepper to taste

Instructions:

- Steam broccoli until tender-crisp.
- Toss onion and garlic in hot olive oil for 5 minutes, or until softened.
- Add broth, milk, and steamed veggies to the pan.
- Simmer for 5 minutes.
- Blend the soup smoothly using an immersion blender or in batches in a regular blender.
- Return soup to pot and stir in cheddar cheese until melted.
- Season with salt and pepper to taste.

Bone-loving benefits: Broccoli is a treasure trove of calcium and vitamin C, both important for bone development. Cheddar cheese adds a large amount of calcium and protein, improving your skeletal system.

Lentil and Walnut Salad with Lemon Vinaigrette:

Ingredients:

- 1 cup cooked lentils (brown or green)
- 1/2 cup chopped walnuts
- 1 cup mixed greens
- 1/4 cup diced red onion
- 1/4 cup crumbled feta cheese
- 2 tbsp olive oil
- 1 tbsp lemon juice
- 1 tsp Dijon mustard
- Salt and pepper to taste

Instructions:

- Combine lentils, peanuts, leaves, and onion in a bowl.
- Whisk together olive oil, lemon juice, Dijon mustard, salt, and pepper for a dressing.
- Coat the salad with dressing and toss.
- Top with crumbled feta cheese.

Bone-loving benefits: Lentils are rich in iron and plant-based protein, important for bone health. Walnuts add omega-3 fatty acids, known to lower inflammation and support bone density. Feta cheese adds another dose of calcium and protein for a well-rounded bone-building boost.

Foods that support cardiovascular health and reduce inflammation

Mediterranean Salmon with Lemon-Garlic Spinach and Roasted Sweet Potatoes:

Ingredients:

- Salmon slices (4)
- Olive oil
- Garlic cloves (minced)
- Lemon juice
- Sea salt and black pepper
- Fresh spinach
- Sweet potatoes (diced)
- Cherry tomatoes (halved)
- Kalamata olives (sliced)
- Feta cheese (crumbled)

Instructions:

- Preheat oven to 400°F. Coat sweet potatoes and tomatoes with olive oil, season with salt and pepper, and roast for 20 minutes.
- While potatoes cook, marinate salmon in olive oil, garlic, lemon juice, salt, and pepper for 15 minutes.
- Sauté spinach until softened.
- Pan-fry or bake salmon until cooked through.

- Assemble the dish with cooked veggies, wilted spinach, fish, olives, and feta cheese.

Cardiovascular Benefits: This dish is packed with heart-healthy omega-3s from salmon, fiber from sweet potatoes, and vitamins from tomatoes and spinach. Olive oil gives monounsaturated fats, good for cholesterol levels.

Spicy Lentil and Kale Soup with Turmeric:

Ingredients:

- Lentils (rinsed)
- Vegetable broth
- Chopped kale
- Diced carrots and celery
- Onion and garlic (minced)
- Ginger (grated)
- Turmeric powder
- Cumin and cilantro flour
- Black pepper
- Coconut milk (optional, for smooth taste)

Instructions:

- Stir-fry onion and garlic in olive oil until translucent.
- Add carrots, celery, beans, and spices. Saute for a few minutes.

- Pour in broth and bring to a boil, then cook for 30 minutes or until lentils are soft.
- Add kale and cook for 5 more minutes.
- Stir in coconut milk (if using) and adjust spices.

Anti-inflammatory Power: This soup is a powerhouse of anti-inflammatory foods like turmeric, ginger, and kale. Lentils provide protein and fiber, while veggies add vitamins and minerals for general health.

Berry Walnut Overnight Oats:

Ingredients:

- Rolled oats
- Chia seeds
- Greek yogurt
- Milk (cow, plant-based, or plain nut milk)
- Mixed plums
- Chopped walnuts

Instructions:

- Combine oats, chia seeds, yogurt, and milk in a jar or container. Stir in berries and walnuts.
- Refrigerate overnight.
- Enjoy cold in the morning, or warm it up slightly for a cozy breakfast.

Heart-Healthy Goodness: This breakfast offers steady energy from oats and fiber, healthy fats from walnuts, and antioxidants from berries. Greek yogurt provides protein and calcium, important for heart health.

Brain-boosting dishes to improve cognitive function and memory

Mediterranean Memory Salad:

Ingredients:

- Quinoa (cooked)
- Chopped tomatoes, cucumbers, olives, and red onion
- Grilled fish or tofu (cubed)
- Feta cheese (crumbled)
- Dried oregano and thyme
- Extra virgin olive oil
- Lemon juice

Instructions:

- Combine rice, veggies, protein, and cheese in a bowl.
- Drizzle with olive oil and lemon juice.
- Sprinkle with oregano and thyme.
- Enjoy the cool crunch and brain-boosting effects!

Nutrients: This salad is a symphony of omega-3 fatty acids from salmon/tofu, antioxidants from the veggies, and choline from eggs (which can be added), important for memory and brain function. Quinoa provides B vitamins for energy and healthy brain function, while olive oil's healthy fats feed neurons.

Turmeric-Tastic Lentil Curry:

Ingredients:

- Brown beans (rinsed)
- Coconut juice
- Chopped carrots, potatoes, and spinach
- Diced onion and garlic
- Grated ginger and turmeric
- Garam masala and cumin
- Cilantro (chopped)

Instructions:

- Sauté onion and garlic.
- Add spices, ginger, and turmeric.
- Stir in beans, veggies, and coconut milk.
- Simmer until lentils are tender.
- Garnish with parsley before serving.

Nutrients: Curcumin in turmeric boasts anti-inflammatory qualities, protecting brain cells and possibly slowing cognitive decline. Lentil's plant-based protein and iron improve blood flow to the brain, while spinach offers brain-protective Vitamin K.

Chocolate-Cherry Overnight Oats:

Ingredients:

- Rolled oats

- Plant-based milk (unsweetened)
- Chia seeds
- Cocoa powder
- Chopped nuts or seeds
- Cherries (sweet or tart)

Instructions:

- Mix oats, milk, chia seeds, and cocoa powder in a jar.
- Refrigerate overnight.
- Top with nuts/seeds and cherries in the morning.

Nutrients: Dark chocolate's flavanols improve blood flow and memory, while fiber-rich oats keep you feeling refreshed and focused. Chia seeds and nuts offer omega-3s and B vitamins, further boosting brain health. Tart cherries, rich in antioxidants, help fight free radicals that hurt brain cells.

Mood-enhancing meals to combat stress and anxiety

Sunshine Salmon with Lemon-Herb Zest:

Ingredients:

- Salmon fillets
- Olive oil
- Garlic and ginger (minced)
- Fresh herbs (dill, parsley, basil)
- Lemon zest and juice
- Honey
- Roasted veggies (broccoli, asparagus, or zucchini)

Instructions:

- Preheat oven to 400°F. Toss veggies with olive oil and cook until tender.
- Combine olive oil, garlic, ginger, herbs, lemon zest juice, and honey in a bowl. Coat salmon fillets with the mixture.
- Place salmon on a baking sheet and roast alongside vegetables for 15-20 minutes, or until cooked through.

Mood Boosters: Omega-3 fatty acids in salmon are brain powerhouses, supporting cognitive function and reducing anxiety. Vitamin C from lemon promotes dopamine production, a natural mood elevator. Herbs like dill and parsley are rich in B vitamins, crucial for stress management and nervous system health.

Zesty Quinoa Power Bowl with Tahini Dressing:

Ingredients:

- Cooked quinoa
- Roasted chickpeas (seasoned with paprika and cayenne pepper)
- Chopped cucumbers, tomatoes, and radishes
- Crumbled feta cheese
- Tahini dressing (tahini, lemon juice, water, garlic, olive oil)
- Fresh mint or cilantro

Instructions:

- Combine cooked quinoa, chickpeas, vegetables, and feta cheese in a bowl.
- Stir-fry onion and garlic in olive oil until translucent.

Mood Boosters: Quinoa is a protein and fiber powerhouse, keeping you feeling full and your energy stable. Hummus and tahini dressing are fantastic sources of tryptophan, converted to mood-regulating serotonin in the body. Spicy notes from cayenne pepper can activate endorphins, natural stress-fighters.

Dark Chocolate & Banana Overnight Oats:

Ingredients:

- Rolled oats
- Almond milk (or your preferred milk)
- Chia seeds
- Greek yogurt
- Mashed banana
- Cocoa powder
- Dark chocolate chips (optional)

Instructions:

- Combine oats, milk, chia seeds, yogurt, banana, and cocoa powder in a jar or container. Stir well.
- Refrigerate for 4+ hours, preferably overnight. Top with dark chocolate chips for a decadent treat.

Mood Boosters: Bananas are rich in potassium, vital for blood pressure regulation and stress reduction. Dark chocolate with at least 70% cocoa contains flavanols, powerful antioxidants that improve blood flow and brain function, promoting calmness. Magnesium in nuts and seeds aids muscle relaxation and sleep, key allies in anxiety management.

Chapter 7: The Joy of Cooking: Tips, Tricks, and Kitchen Magic

Meal planning and prep strategies for busy lives

Ah, the busy life. Work deadlines, school runs, social commitments – where does the time for healthy, delicious meals even fit in? Enter the culinary superpower known as meal planning and prep. No longer the domain of Pinterest perfectionists, this strategy is for anyone who values good food without the daily kitchen scramble.

Planning Your Culinary Conquest:

- Get Calendar Cozy: Start by mapping out your week. Identify busy nights and potential leftover-friendly days. Plan simpler meals around hectic schedules and save more elaborate dishes for calmer evenings.
- Theme Nights are Fun: Mexican Mondays, Taco Tuesdays, Wholesome Wednesdays – designate themes to spark inspiration and prevent mealtime monotony.
- Double Up the Goodness: Cook larger batches of grains, proteins, or roasted vegetables in advance.

They become building blocks for multiple meals, saving you time and effort.

- Shop Smart, Not Scattered: Make a list based on your plan and stick to it! Avoid impulse buys and ensure you have everything you need to conquer the week's meals.

Prepping like a Pro:

- Chop Once, Eat Twice: Dice onions, peppers, and herbs on a designated prep day. These prepped veggies instantly elevate salads, stir-fries, and omelets throughout the week.
- Portion Perfection: Divide cooked grains, proteins, and sauces into individual containers for grab-and-go lunches or quick dinner reheats.
- Mason Jar Magic: Layer overnight oats, salads, or mason jar meals for portable lunches or light dinners. They're delicious, visually appealing, and require minimal assembly.
- Freezer is Your Friend: Soups, stews, and even some cooked grains freeze beautifully. Batch cook on a weekend and enjoy healthy, homemade meals on busy weeknights.
- Tools of the Trade:
- Invest in good storage containers: Airtight containers keep food fresh and prevent freezer burn. Look for compartmentalized options for portion control.

- Embrace the reusable revolution: Ditch plastic wrap and single-use bags. Silicone lids, reusable food wraps, and cloth napkins are eco-friendly and efficient.
- Befriend your freezer: Invest in freezer bags and portioned containers to maximize freezing potential.
- Apps galore: There are countless meal planning and grocery list apps out there. Find one that suits your style and use it to streamline the process.

Remember: Meal planning and prep is not about rigid rules or Instagram-worthy perfection. It's about finding a system that works for you, saving you time, and ensuring you eat well even on the busiest days. Experiment, adapt, and most importantly, have fun! So, conquer the kitchen chaos, embrace the joy of planning, and enjoy the peace of mind that comes with knowing you have delicious, healthy meals at your fingertips every night.

Creative substitutions and pantry staples for versatile cooking

Let's face it, unexpected recipe changes can throw even the most seasoned chef off balance. A missing ingredient, a forgotten grocery run, or simply a desire to experiment – these are all opportunities to unleash your inner culinary MacGyver! Here's a guide to navigating kitchen challenges with clever substitutions and pantry staples for versatile cooking:

The Art of Substitution:

- Vegetable Chameleon: Out of broccoli for your stir-fry? Zucchini, green beans, or even thinly sliced cabbage can step in as worthy replacements, offering similar textures and nutritional benefits.
- The Power of Powder: Fresh herbs wilting? Don't fret! Dried herbs, though slightly concentrated in flavor, can be your savior. Use half the quantity of dried herbs compared to fresh for a balanced taste.
- Missing the Main Event: Protein swap alert! Ground turkey can often stand in for ground beef in chili or meatballs, offering a leaner alternative. Tofu cubes can mimic chicken in stir-fries, while lentils or beans can bulk up soups and stews.
- Dairy Dilemmas: No worries if you're out of milk! Broth or even unsweetened coconut milk can work wonders in creamy sauces and soups. For baking, consider applesauce or mashed bananas as egg substitutes, or try flaxseed "eggs" made with ground flaxseed and water for vegan baking adventures.

Pantry Powerhouses:

- Beans, the Marvelous Multitaskers: Canned beans are affordable, shelf-stable, and oh-so-versatile. From creamy hummus dips to hearty salads, bean burgers, and protein-packed pasta sauces, the possibilities are endless.

- Rice, the Reassuring Reinforcer: Brown rice, quinoa, or even couscous can swap in for traditional white rice, adding fiber and nutrients to your meals. Leftovers? Get creative! Turn them into fried rice, stuffed peppers, or even breakfast porridge.
- The Mighty Magic of Spices: Herbs and spices like paprika, cumin, turmeric, and chili flakes can instantly transform the flavor profile of your dish. Experiment with different combinations to create unique and exciting culinary journeys.
- Pasta's Playful Possibilities: Fusilli, penne, spaghetti – while familiar shapes are comforting, don't underestimate the joy of experimenting! Rotini's twists hold sauce beautifully, while orecchiette's little shells cradle hearty toppings. Explore different shapes and textures to make mealtimes more fun.

Beyond the Recipe:

- Embrace Seasonality: Let fresh, local produce guide your cooking. Seasonal vegetables are often at their peak flavor and affordability, offering endless inspiration for creative substitutions.
- Leftovers, Reworked: Don't relegate leftovers to the back of the fridge! Get creative! Leftover roasted chicken can become a nourishing salad

topping, while cooked quinoa can be transformed into veggie fritters or breakfast porridge.
- Small Tweaks, Big Impact: A splash of lemon juice, a handful of chopped nuts, or a sprinkle of fresh herbs can elevate a simple dish into a culinary masterpiece. Big results often start with tiny tweaks.

So, the next time a missing ingredient or a culinary whim sparks your imagination, remember – with a little creativity and these versatile pantry staples, you can conquer the kitchen and turn any meal into a delicious adventure!